I0415545

Start Living Gluten Free

A Beginners Guide to a Gluten Free Diet

by Simone Donovan
http://simonedonovan.com/

Copyright © 2013

Other Books From This Author

The In's and Out's of Coconut Oil: A Beginners Guide

Modern Paleo Book 1: A Beginners Guide to the Paleo Diet

Modern Paleo Book 2: An Athletic Approach To The Paleo Diet

Book Bundles:

In's and Out's of Coconut Oil and Modern Paleo Beginner's Guide Book Bundle

Modern Paleo Book Bundle

The In's and Out's of Coconut Oil, Modern Paleo The Beginner's Guide and Athletic Approach Book Bundle

Simone Donovan
http://simonedonovan.com/

Start Living Gluten Free

Contents

Start Living Gluten Free

Introduction

There is lots of talk about Gluten these days in the media, health food circles and online forums regarding its impact on your health and its necessity in the foods that people consume on a day to day basis.

Less than a decade ago, most people had no idea what Gluten even was, unless they already suffered from celiac disease, or an allergic reaction to its involvement in their diets. Now, thousands and thousands of food labels on the market state proudly that they are "Gluten Free!"

Although this statement is popular, it is not required by the law in the UK or the USA to be listed on labels. In the UK, it is only the requirement that it is listed on cereals, but other products are completely voluntary, and up to the manufacturer or distributor. In the United States, the United States Food and Drug Administration (USFDA) do not require its labeling at all, as it is considered GRAS – generally regarded as safe.

Although a number of companies have taken the lead in adding the labeling to their foods as a result of the popular switch in the states to the gluten free lifestyle. Canada, however, has jumped ahead of the curve and requires clear gluten labeling on all foods that include gluten "at a level greater than 10 ppm."

The truth is, Gluten, as it will be explained in detail below, exists in a lot of products naturally, and is used as an additive in countless others. If you are allergic to gluten you already know the dangers of eating it – just as anyone with a food allergy is aware when they consume the foods that are off limits to their system.

Celiac Disease, which is the autoimmune disease that requires a gluten free diet, otherwise the result is severe damage to the intestines and the body's ability to consume nutrients, is a very serious condition that must be maintained at all times. Even consuming foods with latent gluten additives can cause severe pain and undesirable results, while causing permanent damage.

There are others who may not have the disease, but are simply sensitive to gluten – or gluten intolerable, which results in pain and discomfort as well, leading them to avoid gluten-laced foods at all times.

These two conditions are clear, and will be explained in detail throughout the book. However, it begs the question: What happened to the rest of the world? Why did everyone become adverse to Gluten in the same time frame, and what exactly did it do to everyone to make them so anti-gluten? Was it just a matter of diagnosing the root of their ills? Or is it simply a drive to be more health conscious, and maintaining an accurate count of what they putting into their bodies?

From genetically modified organisms, which are the new talk of the town, to organic produce and its relative involvement in allergy symptoms, people are finally paying attention to the foods they eat. This is great news, especially when you can control your diet by shopping for safe and tasty foods, and not simply given less than healthy options as sustenance. For the sake of staying on topic, and not debating unhealthy eating options as a whole, let's jump right in to the Gluten-ness facts.

Chapter One

Gluten Free

What is gluten?

Gluten is a hidden gem in a number of foods that no one knew they loved. It is the substance that makes dough rise and keep its elasticity, while providing that delicious chewy texture that the world thought came naturally. Honestly, it is natural in these cases, and is specifically regarded as a protein composite processed from wheat, barley and rye.

It exists in everything from pizza dough to salad dressing and soups and crackers. Once you understand how many things gluten actually exists in, it will become clear why the gluten free packaging has become so popular.

Going gluten free

If you currently suffer from celiac disease, which one in 133 individuals are suggested to –

which is up from the one in ten thousand that was believed only a decade ago, you absolutely should already be eating a gluten free diet. The fact is, if you suffer from this disease, you will not only feel the repercussions through upset stomach symptoms and enflamed intestines, but you are falling victim to the damages of those two organs that may result in infertility, osteoporosis and intestinal cancer.

In fact not everyone who avoids Gluten has celiac disease, but there is a heightened negative response referred to as non-celiac gluten sensitivity that causes stomach cramps, bloating and diarrhea, but does not result in damage to the actual intestines – just absolute discomfort. Absolute discomfort may be enough for the 20 million projected sufferers to kick the additive from their diet. Similar to those who cannot eat spicy foods, or certain styles of foods without feelings the physical effects, gluten sensitive people are going to know the minute they digest foods that contain gluten, and it is not going to make for a pleasant evening.

For both parties, the bad news is, even with the emergence of gluten free labeling, kicking gluten completely takes serious commitment. It takes patience, perseverance and focus, as gluten can hide in just about anything. This means never walking to a co-workers candy dish and simply popping the contents inside into your mouth. You are going to have to consciously think about everything you eat going forward, and quite honestly – that is not a bad thing.

Where is it found?

The better question might be "where isn't it found?" Although they may be a broad and sweeping statement, the hard truth is that most breads and bread flours are high in gluten. As mentioned previously, it allows the yeast to rise and promotes elasticity - so your pizza dough is easily spread for baking, and your homemade rolls rise to perfect. It also gives the chewiness and moisture component a boost, so you are in heaven with every crumby bite of baguette you ingest. If breads were the only source of gluten, it would be a lot easier to kick than it actually is, and would promote the renewed popularity of the Atkins Diet.

However, it is also in imitation meats, which are big on the vegetarian and vegan circuit, and allows the foods to soak up the broth they are cooked in to become firm and moist. Some of the hidden, so to speak, gluten infused foods can include everything from beer to soy sauce and ice cream to ketchup. The list, quite honestly, is endless in this category, which is why labeling has become so popular - and in the case of those who suffer physically from eating gluten - necessary.

Common, gluten-infused foods include:

- Bagels
- Beer
- Bread
- Cakes and pies
- Candies
- Cereals
- Coffee Substitutes
- Cookies and Crackers
- Croutons
- Condiments (Most!)
- French Fries
- Gravies
- Imitation Meat or Seafood
- Licorice
- Malt
- Matzo
- Oats
- Pasta
- Pizza
- Pretzels

- Processed Meat (Hot Dogs, Sausages and Lunch Meat)
- Salad Dressings
- Sauces
- Seasoned Rice Mixes
- Seasoned Snack Foods (Potato and Tortilla Chips)
- Self-basting Poultry
- Soups and Soup Bases
- Vegetables in Sauce

This certainly is NOT the entire list. There are thousands of foods that contain gluten, and if you are serious about ejecting it from your diet, you really have to pay attention to the food you eat. This means reading labels, doing research and cooking with all natural ingredients that are not going to leave you with an upset stomach later.

The good news is, fresh foods including vegetables and fruits straight from your produce stand do not contain gluten. As with just about everything else, the more natural the food's composition, the less likely it is to contain gluten. That is why you typically only see the words "Gluten Free!" on packaging, because the foods are packaged – and not naturally found in the world.

The oldest rule in dieting is to steer clear of processed and packaged foods. Items that exist in your freezer section are almost always the highest in calorie, fat and sodium content, and are almost always loaded with gluten to help the "bonding" of the food. When you steer clear of these foods altogether, you have literally decreased your gluten intake by twenty five percent.

The benefits of gluten free eating

Although gluten itself is not particularly "bad" for you, unless you have an affliction to its existence, there are benefits to cutting it out of your diet. For instance, salad dressing has always been bad for you, no matter who you are, even if all you consume day in and day out is salads. It is just a terrible condiment, as is mayonnaise, which also contains gluten and should have been cut from your diet long ago.

Going gluten free means passing up all of the unhealthy elements that you have always wanted to cut from your diet to begin with. For instance, if you have always known that you should order your salads with the dressing on the side - or without it at all - but still ate the meal when it came poured over the top of it, going gluten free will lead you to enforce those requests. In fact, you should not even have the salad dressing served on the side, as they usually place the small open containers inside the salad, causing spillage on its way out of the kitchen.

And the next time you ask for no salad dressing and your salad arrives drowned in the creamy substance, you are going to have to send it back. This is what a gluten free lifestyle means - taking no chances in consuming the ingredient.

Overall, this is great news! If you are going gluten free for health reasons, and not because you have celiac disease or are sensitive to it, you are going to cut so many unhealthy additives from your diet immediately that you will begin feeling better right away!

Here are a few quick nutritional notes, as a common condiment application, and how it affects your calorie, fat and sodium intake. What you thought was a harmless application before is going to be clearly detrimental to your dieting efforts now.

Ranch dressing and mayonnaise(Real & Miracle Whip) nutritional values

Ranch Dressing
Serving Size: Two Tablespoons
Calories: 148
Calories from Fat: 130
Fat: 15.6 grams (nearly a quarter of your recommended daily intake!)
Saturated Fat: 2.4 grams
Cholesterol: 8 milligrams
Sodium: 287 milligrams

There is no vitamin content, and it registers with a grade of D- with nutritionists. When you get rid of gluten, you also say goodbye to these empty calories, which is a HUGE benefit to your nutritional intake – especially when you stop drowning all of the nutrients of your salad with this awful topping.

Hellman's "Real" Mayonnaise
Serving Size: 13 grams, which equals almost .46 ounces, or close to ONE tablespoon
Calories: 90
Calories from Fat: 90
Fat: 10 grams (15% of your recommended daily intake!)
Saturated Fat: 1.5 grams
Cholesterol: 5 milligrams
Sodium: 75 milligrams

There is not a single drop of nutrition that exists in this product. They claim the contents are made from eggs, vinegar and oils, but at no time do they explain what the added flavors are, but they are required to list – for the record – that it is "not a significant source of dietary fiber, sugars, vitamin A, vitamin C, calcium or iron." That, quite honestly, says enough.

Miracle Whip (Characterized as "Salad Dressing" and "Mayonnaise")

Serving Size: 15 grams
Calories: 40
Calories from Fat: 31
Fat: 3.5grams
Saturated Fat: .5 grams
Cholesterol: 5 milligrams
Sodium: 120 milligrams

Although Miracle Whip is not as bad as real mayonnaise, consider the fact that 15 grams is less than a spread across a normal sized piece of bread. And then consider how many times you would apply it to your sandwich before making the switch to gluten free eating. Since you will be giving both up with your new gluten free diet, you are saving yourself a ton of bad consumption values, and that makes for a healthier you every day of the week.

Chapter Two

Overview of the Health Benefits

Is it bad for me?

In a word, no. It is not "bad" for you per se, unless you have celiac disease or an uncomfortable reaction to gluten laced foods. If you can eat a sandwich on a hearty loaf of bread with no trouble, or enjoy a beer or a bagel without any discomfort, you are probably fine to eat whatever you want that includes gluten. However, giving up gluten does require that you give up a lot of unhealthy, processed foods.

It is always healthier to eat foods that do not come wrapped in plastic or cardboard. The dead truth about packaged foods, for the most part, is that they are processed – which is bad for you. Not only do they contain gluten, but they contain preservatives, dyes and things you cannot pronounce. Going gluten free means giving up these other terrible additives too, for the most part, and it may help your digestive system take a break from the hard to process foods you have been feeding it all of these years.

Gluten free also means no fried foods. No heavy breading or French fries, which is a great way to cut those disgusting, unhealthy foods that cause heart disease and high blood pressure from your diet. So when you think of all the foods that typically contain gluten, it may be true that it IS bad for you! To avoid contradiction, it is fair to say that gluten – as it exists naturally – is not bad for you. However, the foods it is commonly associated with it usually are.

Is gluten free healthy for everyone?

Gluten free living is perfectly healthy, as long as you are supplementing your whole grain intake along the way. Your digestive health will improve, and allow your body to process the vitamins and minerals you are eating with greater success. This means you will begin building healthy muscles that burn fat as energy. Your digestive system will be able to process foods cleanly, which means you are ridding the body of waste more efficiently, and keeping a proper balance of good and bad bacteria in your gut – boosting your immune system.

The health benefits

There are several things you need to know about going gluten free, as it is not as simple as just giving up bread. There are many health benefits that can be enjoyed from cutting the overly processed foods that gluten hides in from your diet, but there are also a few foods that have tremendous nutritional value that coincidentally contain gluten. It seems confusing at first glance, but you will get the hang of it.

This eBook is designed specifically to outline the facts behind gluten free living, so you can make informed decisions about the foods you eat. After all, that is the largest component of accessing and maintaining a healthy diet, being informed about the ingredients and what they mean to your body's overall health.

With that said it is important to know that foods that are billed as gluten free are not necessarily healthier. They can still be high in calories and fat, so keep an eye on the labels of the food you eat (this will be discussed in detail in an upcoming chapter), so you are not simply substituting your current unhealthy choices for gluten free foods that are just as unhealthy. This is important distinction.

Gluten free does not mean fat free, additive or preservative free: It simply means that there is no wheat, barley, malt, oats or rye in its make-up. It cannot be overstated enough that gluten free foods are not diet foods, necessarily.

When you practice the diet correctly, you will be eliminating fried foods from your diet because of their gluten laden breading, as well as food that are high sugar like cookies, cakes and pastries. With those eliminations, you are already on your way to being a healthier human being. Kicking these gluten-laced foods are something everyone should do, just to keep your health in check as a whole, so the benefits will make themselves known rather quickly.

Some of the other health benefits of going gluten free can include:

- Boost to the Digestive Health
- Improved Cholesterol Levels
- Increased Energy Levels
- Lessen Cancer Risks
- Lower the Risk of Diabetes
- Protecting Your Body from Viruses & Germs
- Reduce the Risk of Heart Disease

When you choose to go gluten free, you will eat

more fruits and vegetables, boosting your natural vitamin, mineral and anti-oxidant intake, which allows you to be healthier internally. This is the key to most dieting tactics: The better you eat, the better you will feel, and your health will follow suit. Going gluten free is not any different.

When you are adding better foods to your diet, your body can eliminate waste easier, while clearing the way for your digestive system to absorb all of the good nutrients as a result. It is, as they say, a win/win!

Gluten free vs. Grain free

With the gluten free craze in full swing, some doctors warn that individuals are giving up the healthy whole grains they need to maintain a balanced diet as a result of giving up breads and cereals. This does not have to be the case, but it will take an effort to find the grains you can eat to balance out your diet, while remaining gluten free.

Whole grains are rich in vitamins and minerals, especially iron and B vitamins. In fact the Dietary Guidelines for Americans states that half of all their carbohydrate intake should come from whole grain products. Whole grains are a tremendous source of fiber, as well, so incorporating them into your diet while going gluten free should be maintained.

In order to do so, you will have to concentrate on the whole grains that do NOT contain gluten. Researching your favorite grains will help – as wheat, barley, rye, malt and even oats (per some doctor's recommendations) are off limits. If you have concerns about removing these items from your diet safely, talk to your doctor about the safe alternatives that will help you maintain a gluten free diet. They may be able to give you some brand name foods that will help you distinguish between what you can and cannot eat going forward.

Some great sources of whole grains that are gluten free include:

- Amaranth
- Buckwheat
- Corn and Cornmeal
- Job's Tears
- Millet
- Montina
- Quinoa
- Rice
- Sorghum
- Soy
- Teff
- Wild Rice

Check your local whole foods stores and nutrition outlets for gluten free whole grains that are nutritious and filling, without interrupting your gluten free approach to dieting. Also, online gluten free stores are excited to show off their wares, including gluten free cereals and breads that taste just like the real thing.

Changing your approach to food

One of the best things about changing your diet to go gluten free is that you are going to have to change your approach to how and what you eat altogether. Thinking about what you eat, before you eat it, is the best way to avoid hazardous foods with high fat content and sodium.

Consider this scenario: Before you go gluten free, it would probably take no time to sit down at a restaurant and enjoy a basket of French fries with friends. If someone orders an appetizer, and you are joining them, it takes zero thought to grab a small plate and enjoy the offering alongside the rest of the group. Even people who are on low fat diets, or who are following a dieting regimen like the South Beach Diet or the Flat Belly Diet will splurge on an order of cheese fries or fried mushrooms with friends from time to time.

When dieting, eating a single fried pickle or zucchini is not going to blow your entire weight loss plan out of the water. It is simply considered a treat, and not something you would eat regularly, so what's the big deal?

The big deal is that when you have an aversion to gluten, whether it is sensitivity or diagnosed celiac disease, the consequences of sharing that same appetizer can be grave. When you give up gluten, you must think about everything you ingest to avoid discomfort and possibly painful and health injuring side effects. Even if you were safely able to eat these foods before, it is the perfect lifestyle to help you avoid them going forward, which exactly what giving up gluten is: a lifestyle.

If you are giving up gluten for the sake of eating healthier, that is a fantastic start. However, you are going to have to approach the diet as if eating gluten will physically harm you - like those who have a true aversion to it do. When you do, you can avoid numerous unhealthy food options while plying your system with only the best nutritional options available.

You will be amazed at the boost to your health, which will only encourage you to continue on a gluten free path.

Adapting to gluten free eating

Because of the popularity of gluten free eating, adapting to the diet is going to take more discipline on your part than it does searching for available foods. As more and more people turn to a healthier eating pattern there are online groups, forums and even recipes that allow you to enjoy a gluten free lifestyle while still eating the delicious foods that you love.

When you are inside of your home, you can control all of your own ingredients and food handling responsibilities, so in order to adapt a gluten free diet you may have to prepare your own meals for a while, until you get the hang of what you can and cannot eat. Making your own lunch, for instance, is a great way to eat healthier at the office. This is a perfect approach for any diet, as you can keep you calorie count down, while packing only the foods you like instead of leaving your meals to chance.

When you switch to a gluten free diet, you can pack only those items that fall within its guidelines, and feel good about the things you are eating as a result. This will give you plenty of time to scan the internet, as well, for gluten free food alternatives, since you are having lunch at your desk.

Ride the popularity of this dieting approach and stock up on gluten free foods that your entire family will enjoy. A word to the wise, however, is to purchase these items with regularity, without pointing them out to your children (if you have children). Whenever kids feel like they are being deprived of something, they want it more. Treat this transition as a normal evolution to eating healthier, and not as a stripping away of all things they love.

In addition, talk to other adults about your gluten free lifestyle. Your friends and family should know that you are going gluten free, if they do not already, so they can accommodate you at dinners, or generally accept the fact that you are going to bring foods to pitch ins that are gluten free. Getting the support you need to remain gluten free will help you feel satisfied with your decision.

Just as it is with any other diet, when others know your eating habits they are more likely to support your choices by picking restaurants that cater to your needs. Likewise, you can enjoy a healthy social life as a result, instead of hiding at your desk each time the rest of your coworkers are heading to lunch. Going gluten free is no reason to ostracize yourself from friends or family.

It is a perfect opportunity to explain your motives, and answer any questions they might have about your decision. Who knows? You could help someone else in your group diagnose the root of their digestive discomfort as a result. At no time is this diet going to harm you, especially if you are getting whole grains from other, safe sources, so there is nothing to hide from when others inquire about your motives to go gluten free.

Gluten free family eating(Gluten free with children)

Bringing a gluten free diet into your home is a great way to keep your children healthy, while maintaining their weight. Going gluten free means no more fried foods or unhealthy snacks after school. Again, making a big deal out of the fact that you are going gluten free will only draw their attention to it, leading them (the children, that is) to psychosomatically believe that the foods they are eating taste different, or that they are inferior in taste, texture and quality. This is not true, and although adults are aware of it, children tend to rebel in the food department, especially when change is on the horizon.

There are few easy switches that you can make to keep your kids from making the ever dreaded "I'm not eating *that*!" remarks. First, swap the bread in your home with wheat and gluten free options. There is even a gluten free white bread, if they are already protesting the previous switch to wheat bread that you tried with the last healthy overhaul of your kitchen. It is usually made with potato, instead of wheat, and is just as delicious.

Swap their cereals for corn and rice based options, making sure they do not contain malt for adding flavoring. Larger companies are following the popular suit of labeling their foods as gluten free, so check the cereal aisle thoroughly when you are shopping for the little ones.

Skip the pastas and focus on rice and potatoes. This will be a great change of pace in your home, and will allow all of those empty calories to go by the wayside. In addition, everyone will feel less bloated after a large meal, which is never the case when spaghetti or lasagna is part of the menu. Rice, vegetables and fruits can all be prepared effortlessly, and allow your kids to enjoy foods that are really good for them without spending the entire evening in the kitchen.

One great suggestion is to allow the kids to help in the fruit preparation by using a melon baller, so the fruits are fun to create and eat. If there is a vegetable they like more than others, serve it often. Do not inject spinach into the mix if they never liked it to begin with, as the resistance to going gluten free will only grow.

Stick with what you know, even if that means potatoes eight ways to Sunday, until they are open to trying different foods. Another option would be to let them accompany you to the market, and pick a new fruit or vegetable of their choice for an upcoming meal. This provides the children with ownership over their eating options, and opens their minds to new foods.

Although not all of their choices are going to be stellar, encourage them to try and try again, exploring fruits and vegetables from around the world. A great exercise is to pick a fruit or vegetable from the market, and have the child (age withstanding, of course) research where it grows and when it is in season. This heightens the overall experience, and allows you to add more and more gluten free meal options to the dinner table as a result.

Finally, grille your foods as often as possible - even if you have to use an indoor version of a grilling device (these exist in every size, shape and watt variety imaginable). Whether you are eating chicken, beef or fish, cook it on the grille to maintain a healthier approach to eating. Fried foods are completely out with a gluten free diet, and that is the best thing you can ban in your home while helping your kids appreciate the taste and texture of grilled foods.

This will encourage them to make smart decisions outside of the home as well, and avoid going to for a deep fried chicken sandwich, picking the grilled alternative instead.

Gluten free flavors

This category is a little tougher than most, because it is really hard to purchase seasonings and extracts that are certain to be gluten free. However, some companies have jumped on the popularity bandwagon of gluten free labeling, making it a little easier to procure the spices and flavors you need to season steaks or dry rub a roasted chicken.

There is no actual list of "flavors" necessarily that can be listed with surety. However, check with your local health food stores for seasoning alternatives, and online outlets for oils, extracts and sauces that are made from all natural ingredients that are also gluten free.

You may find that sticking with your produce section will get you everything you need, including fresh rosemary and lemons for chicken seasoning, and sea salt and cracked pepper for steaks.

Expectations

Depending on your reasons for going gluten free, your expectations may differ. If you are suffering from gluten sensitivity or celiac disease, the expectation is that you are going to begin feeling less bloated, uncomfortable, and outright ill from avoiding gluten as a whole. This expectation is correct. If gluten is physically making you sick, avoiding it will help you feel healthier, with better digestion and less gastrointestinal problems. It will also help you restore the nutrient levels your body needs to actively enjoy life.

If you are giving up gluten with the expectation of losing weight, you may be surprised by the outcome. First, giving up gluten will cut a lot of unhealthy foods from your consumption options. This is a great way to get your healthy eating habits kick started. So if you consume a submarine sandwich every day, and stop to follow a gluten free diet, then yes – you will probably lose weight pretty quickly.

However, if you are already eating a balanced diet, removing gluten is only going to supplement your current eating habits for the better. You will not, however, drop a lot of weight as a result. The same goes for fried foods. If you are currently eating them daily, and give them up as part of your gluten free lifestyle, you will lose weight. These scenarios are less about giving up gluten, necessarily, as they are about giving up the things you should already NOT be eating so regularly.

Maintain a positive approach, keep an open mind and be realistic about what a gluten free diet will bring to your life. Although new studies are suggesting that going gluten free can lead directly to weight loss, the findings are inconclusive so far, and are typically the result of the previously mentioned scenarios of giving up the bad foods, and losing the weight and feeling healthier as a result.

Should you go gluten free?

The short answer to "should you go gluten free?" is, why not? As outlined previously, gluten comes in the form of mostly unhealthy foods, with the exception of some whole grains. In fact, you may have already noticed that some of the things you are currently purchasing are already labeled as gluten free. You certainly would not return a bag of tortilla chips to the shelf because they are gluten free, in favor of a full gluten alternative, would you? Let's hope not.

Chapter Three

Gluten Sensitivity and Celiac Disease

Helping with allergies

If you are allergic to gluten, or even sensitive to its intake, going gluten free is going to help you tremendously. A food allergy is a very serious thing, no matter how mild or severe. Some people cannot eat peanuts, or they will go into anaphylactic shock as a result, which can cause death. Others simply cannot eat garlic or onions, lest they want to punish their digestive system with cramping, diarrhea and the possible stripping of nutrients from their body in the process. Food allergies can cause everything from tongue swelling to headaches and rashes to fevers.

Although allergies play a big role in the way people eat, so do their eating habits. If you are a vegetarian and eat meat for the first time in a while, your body is going to reject it, causing serious digestive issues that will not only be uncomfortable, but damaging to the gastrointestinal tract. When you finally get rid of gluten from your diet, chances of reintroducing it will be slim to none, otherwise your body will react poorly. This is good news for giving up fried foods altogether, which is something that no one needs in their diet.

What is gluten sensitivity & intolerance?

Gluten sensitivity and intolerance is much like an allergic reaction, which causes discomfort and digestion problems. Some people experience similar effects when they eat spicy foods or certain items they know their body cannot handle without ravaging the digestive system as a result.

When someone is sensitive or intolerant of gluten, it is not any different from someone who is lactose intolerant drinking a large glass of milk. You can eat the ingredients, but you are going to pay the price for it. Some effects gluten has on those who are sensitive or intolerant include:

- Abdominal Cramping
- Bloating
- Diarrhea
- Flatulence

The difference between sensitivity and intolerance when compared to celiac disease is that there is currently no proof that the previous condition causes damage to the intestinal lining.

What is celiac disease?

Celiac disease is a much more serious condition than sensitivity or intolerance to gluten. When someone with celiac disease ingests gluten their immune system responds by damaging the small intestine.

The small intestine contains tiny, finger like

protrusions called Villi. Villi grab and absorb nutrients so the body can respond in a healthy manner – keeping illnesses at bay, while delivering a healthy overall composition as a result. When individuals with celiac disease eat gluten, it damages the Villi, stripping its ability to function and absorb the nutrients the body needs to protect itself and live healthily. This can cause the sufferer to become malnourished, no matter what they eat going forward – even in large, healthy quantities.

Symptoms of celiac disease

Although celiac disease has some of the same symptoms as sensitivity and intolerance, the overall signs are much more severe, and are much more than an upset, bloated stomach. This disease is very serious, and should be caught at the earliest stages to ensure that the body keeps its internal health in check.

Symptoms and signs of celiac disease include:

- Bloating
- Decreased Appetite
- Floating Stools (bloody or fatty)
- Gas
- Intermittent or Constant Diarrhea
- Nausea and/or Vomiting
- Stomach Pain
- Weight Loss

Long term symptoms are severe and can include:

- Arthritis
- Bruising
- Depression & Anxiety
- Fatigue
- Hair Loss
- Itchy Skin (dermatitis)
- Joint Pain
- Low Bone Density

- Missed Menstrual Periods (in women)
- Mouth Sores
- Neurological Problems
- Seizures
- Tingling in Hands and Feet
- Vitamin Deficiencies

Spotting symptoms in childern

Since the effects of celiac disease can be life altering, the earlier it is diagnosed, the better. Children display symptoms similar to adults, but can be very specific and should be addressed immediately.

Celiac disease symptoms in children include:

- Abdominal Pain & Bloating
- Chronic Constipation
- Chronic Diarrhea (which can be bloody)
- Decreased Appetite
- Failure to Gain Weight
- Fatigue
- Growth Problems
- Irritability
- Vomiting

The condition can also be apparent in teenagers, but it usually is triggered by an emotional event, including injury, illness or the loss of a loved one.

The symptoms in teenagers include:

- Abdominal Pain & Bloating
- Delayed Puberty
- Depression
- Dermatitis (itchy skin rash that resembles poison ivy)
- Diarrhea
- Fatigue
- Growth Problems
- Irritability

- Mouth Sores
- Weight Loss

No matter how old you or a loved one is, if you or they exhibit any of these symptoms, it is important to get tested right away to ensure your health is not compromised in the long term.

Getting tested

In an effort to diagnose the disease, individuals who fear its existence, no matter their age, will begin the process with a blood test. If you are positive for the antibodies that exist in celiac disease, the second step is an upper endoscopy to assess the extent of the damage that has already occurred.

Once you are diagnosed, the doctor will work with you to determine the best diet possible for your condition, which means going gluten free immediately. It cannot be overstated enough that individuals with celiac disease must forgo eating gluten at all costs to avoid the long term damage that accompanies the disease.

After the first couple of months, you will need to meet with your doctor again to assess your diet, and overall condition - possibly undergoing another round of tests. All of this is for your own safety. It is important to note that celiac disease is hereditary, and especially common in first degree relatives. So if you have celiac disease, it will be important to get your children tested early to avoid permanent damage as they grow.

Risks of not going gluten free

If you have celiac disease, and simply continue to eat gluten, you are going to damage your intestines beyond repair. Continuing to consume gluten can lead to:

- Intestinal Cancer (although rare)
- Liver Diseases
- Malnutrition

In children and teens, the disease can stunt growth and delay or shorten puberty. Hair loss and dental problems may also occur among young people who continue to eat gluten. The overall effects of continuing to eat gluten AFTER you have been diagnosed with celiac disease can cause serious injury to your body.

Gluten free & child development

Celiac disease can lead to a number of child development problems, which is why it is so important to test your children as soon as possible, to help avoid some of these life altering issues where possible. Some child development issues that occur in children with celiac disease include:

- Abnormal Blood Studies
- Anemia
- Attention Deficit Hyperactive Disorder (ADHD)
- Autism and Learning Disorders
- Cancer Predisposition in Children
- Chronic Bullous Dermatosis
- Delayed Puberty in Boys
- Delayed Puberty in Girls
- Dermatitis Herpetiformis
- Developmental Delay
- Failure to Thrive and Growth Retardation
- Fecal Occult Blood (Blood found in stool that is not visible to the naked eye)
- Glycogenic Acanthosis
- Hypotonia
- Impaired Antibiotic Absorption
- Irritability

- Juvenile Autoimmune Thyroid Disease
- Juvenile Diabetes Type 1
- Juvenile Idiopathic Arthritis
- Osteopenia
- Rickets
- Short Stature
- Stroke in Childhood

Keeping your children healthy, especially if there is a history of celiac disease in your family, is something you should discuss with your physician during pregnancy. Keeping your finger on the pulse of this disease will help you control it, and treat your children accordingly to avoid prolonged health issues.

Diabetes & the gluten effect on insulin sensitivity

Diabetes and celiac disease are both autoimmune diseases, and are radically tied to one another. In fact, medical experts believe that 10% of diabetics suffer from celiac disease as well. The effects of eating gluten can be hazardous to a diabetics overall health.

Gluten mimics insulin, competing for its receptors. In turn, insulin can only work when it is actually bound to its cell receptor, which means it blocks it otherwise (when confused) and the person's glucose levels spike as a result. With the body realizing the increase in sugar from the glucose spike it usually identifies with newly consumed foods it forgoes the actual digestion and distribution process when food is ingested. This begins the process of fluctuating cortisol levels and insulin resistance that result in a diabetic condition.

Aging and hearth health

As people begin to age, nearly everything within the body slows down. This includes the way they digest food, and how their heart reacts to triglycerides. When you decide to maintain a gluten free diet as you age, you are able to consume the vitamins and minerals you need through your digestive system, promoting health as a result.

In addition, gluten free dieting has been connected to lowered cholesterol levels and overall heart health, so you have nothing to lose by giving your body exactly what it needs to age gracefully and healthily.

Chapter Four

Knowing Your Food

Knowing your ingredients

It is always a great idea to know what you are eating. The problem is, sometimes the packaging can be outright confusing. Reading labels is always a great start, but what happens when you stumble across contents that you cannot pronounce? It happens, and it is usually a sign that you should steer clear of whatever is inside.

For the sake of giving up gluten, there are a few buzz words that you will need to know, simply so you can avoid ingesting them. All of the usual suspects, including wheat, barley and rye are definitely on the "Do Not Eat" list, as are oats and malt. However, there are a few others that hide gluten behind their confusing names, and should be avoided, including:

- Bulgur
- Durum flour
- Farina

- Graham flour
- Kamut
- Semolina
- Spelt
- Triticale

Keep an eye out for these ingredients, no matter how deeply buried they are on the list.

Reading and understanding food labels

Once you begin the habit of reading food labels, you will be more alert and focused on what actually goes into your body, which always makes for a healthier you - assuming you heed the warnings, and do not put the additive filled foods in your cart, whether they are gluten free or not.

Food labels contain the nutritional value of foods, along with a list of ingredients that should be sorted through carefully to ensure you are not consuming any gluten.

Avoid anything with ingredients from the list above, and seek out completely gluten free foods that are labeled accordingly. Although the item may not list any of the common gluten offenders, if it lists that the word "flavor" in the description or any confusing components as follows, do not eat it:

- Food additives, such as malt flavoring, modified food starch and others
- Medications and vitamins that use gluten as a binding agent

The rule of thumb should be, if you do not know, or cannot tell whether or not it contains gluten clearly from the packaging, do not eat it. Find something else that is gluten free, and make a note going forward so you do not waste any time in the market searching for foods. At first you are going to read all of the labels in an attempt to educate yourself on their contents, which is a great exercise. Once you find the things you like, that are gluten free, write them down so you can pick them up without the search the next time you shop.

What to look for to recognize gluten free foods

When it comes to gluten free foods, nearly every manufacturer or packaging company is labeling the safe foods accordingly, with bold fonts that say "Gluten Free" or "Certified Gluten Free Food". Although the packaging is different for every item, when you flip it over to check the ingredients it will either list one of the following items, or will state CONTAINS WHEAT INGREDIENTS as an allergy alert.

For the sake of redundancy, because this is really important, it is clearly not okay to eat wheat. It is also not okay to eat barley, rye, oats or malt. In addition, the confusing wheat labeling can be listed as:

- Bulgur
- Durum Flour
- Farina
- Graham Flour
- Kamut
- Semolina
- Spelt
- Triticale

Foods to avoid

There are some easy foods to spot, which are common gluten-laden products. For instance, you are never going to get to eat pizza. Not unless you call ahead, asking if gluten free is an option (it sometimes is, especially in independently owned restaurants - more on this later).

Common, gluten-infused foods include:

- Bagels
- Beer
- Bread
- Cakes and pies
- Candies
- Cereals
- Coffee Substitutes
- Cookies and Crackers
- Croutons
- Condiments (Most!)
- French Fries
- Gravies
- Imitation Meat or Seafood
- Licorice
- Malt
- Matzo
- Oats
- Pasta
- Pizza
- Pretzels
- Processed Meat (Hot Dogs, Sausages and Lunch Meat)
- Salad Dressings
- Sauces
- Seasoned Rice Mixes
- Seasoned Snack Foods (Potato and Tortilla Chips)
- Self-basting Poultry
- Soups and Soup Bases
- Vegetables in Sauce

Although the list seems lengthy, there are even more foods that you can eat, so do not feel overwhelmed by the list of menu items that you must cross off going forward. There is plenty of delicious foods to be had instead – and your body will thank you for consuming more of them!

Foods that can be eaten

Besides the wheat element, most of your diet will stay the same, assuming you do not use a drive thru as your main source of sustenance. Allowed foods, besides the ones labeled as gluten free, include:

- Beans, Seeds, Nuts in their Natural, Unprocessed Form
- Fresh Eggs
- Fresh Meats, Fish and Poultry (not breaded, batter-coated or marinated)
- Fruits and Vegetables
- Most Dairy Products

Whole grain products that are allowed

- Amaranth
- Arrowroot
- Buckwheat
- Corn and Cornmeal
- Flax
- Gluten-free Flours (rice, soy, corn, potato, bean)
- Hominy (corn)
- Millet
- Quinoa
- Rice
- Sorghum
- Soy
- Tapioca
- Teff

Alcohol

Alcohol becomes a tricky point of contention for some nutritionists. First, beer is always out. The malt, barley and wheat that are used in just about every beer on the market, even micro-brews and craft beers, make for a gluten haven. Steer clear of any beer, until you locate the gluten free alternative.

Other liquors are where the contention lies, as some believe that all distilled liquors, even ones with the word "rye" in their name. Theoretically, if the distillation process is done properly, all of the gluten will be removed. However, some whiskey companies add "mash" afterwards, which heightens the color and flavor, which does contain gluten, so it is a tricky concept all around.

To be safe, the Celiac Sprue Association recommends that if you are going to drink – and want to remain gluten free as a result – consume only potato-based vodka, rum and tequila – none of which use grains. If you are going to drink wine or brandy, look for preservative free and dye free options that will allow you to consume them safely from gluten.

Gluten in non food products

Gluten exists in a number of places, and if eating it makes you sick, using the other sources may do the same, especially if it lingers in your toothpaste or Chap Stick. Common non-food products that may contain gluten include:

- Baby Powder
- Bath Salts

- Capsules
- Chewing Gum
- Cleaning Liquids
- Cleaning Liquids
- Communion Wafers
- Conditioner
- Cough Lozenges
- Cough Syrups
- Detergents
- Envelopes
- Latex or Rubber Gloves
- Lip Balm
- Lipstick
- Lotions & Creams
- Make-up
- Mineral Supplements
- Mouthwash
- Paints
- Pet Food
- Pills
- Play Dough
- Shampoo
- Soaps
- Stamps
- Suntan Lotion
- Toothpaste
- Vitamins

If you have questions about any product you use, and whether it contains gluten, do not hesitate to call the manufacturer to find out. This is especially important if you have a child who has a gluten allergy, as kids are constantly putting their fingers and hands in their mouths or on their face. If they are covered in gluten-laden dough or paint, and transferred to their internal organs, the damage is imminent.

Chapter Five

What and Where

Plan ahead

One of the very best ways to maintain a gluten free lifestyle is to plan ahead. Walking into a grocery store without a list is going to take twice as long as if you know exactly which gluten free foods you are going after.

Create a shopping list that contains all of the gluten free foods you need to fill your pantry and refrigerator. If even helps if you list them by brand name - in the case of snacks or treats - so you know exactly which gluten free objects to look for. If you are not sure that a product is gluten free, leave it behind.

Where to shop?

When it comes to shopping for gluten free foods, your local market should suffice. With the popularity of gluten free eating, it is not hard to find everything you might need for your new diet at your local chain grocery store.

However, if you are willing to branch out, and eat whole foods as a result of your new lifestyle change, consider getting your produce from a local farmer's market to ensure its organic growth. Buy your meats, fish and poultry from an actual butcher, instead of at your grocery store – or at the very least look for lean meats at your standard market. Avoid packaged foods as much as possible, and try and shop more often to maintain a fresh approach to eating, while keeping gluten at bay.

If you are looking for spices, rubs or gluten free flavoring additives for your cooking pleasure, stop by your local health food store or nutrition center. If you cannot find what you need on the shelves, ask the person behind the counter if it is available online. Online shopping is a great source for flavors, sauces and spreads that are gluten free, so do not be afraid to experiment.

Keeping within a budget

Going gluten free does not have to break the bank. In fact, the fresher foods are typically less expensive than the packaged ones, and since you are cutting out costly potato chips and frozen pizza snacks, you will have plenty of left over cash for fresh produce and lean meats.

Check your local paper, or look online for coupon savings at your local market. When the gluten free items you love go on sale, buy them in bulk and freeze them! This is especially helpful for chicken, beef or fish.

Shopping and Cooking

Going gluten free requires a change in your lifestyle, not just in your kitchen. You are going to have to change your approach to preparing meals and how you serve foods.

For instance, if everyone in your home is not going gluten free, avoiding cross contamination is going to become an issue. Do you use the same toaster? If so, the gluten laced bread the other person uses is going to remain behind, contaminating your toast as it cooks. Likewise, if the other person uses the peanut butter, regular butter, jams or spreads that you use, chances are they stick a knife in the jar, rub their gluten laced bread, and shove the knife back into the jar. Even though you are using a different knife, the contents of the jar are contaminated.

Avoiding these circumstances takes a lot of foresight, and means scooping the peanut butter from the jar and on to a plate, before spreading it on some gluten-filled bread. It is a lifestyle change, and takes everyone to be on board to ensure there are no incidents of cross contamination.

Once you have sorted out the details, or perhaps have convinced everyone to follow along with the diet (this is best), keep an eye on the utensils you use to prepare foods or to stir pots and pans. When you are ready to start cooking, you will be glad you did!

Adapting Recipes

Listed several times within this eBook are all of the approved gluten free grains and starches you can use to prepare foods. You can still use flour, as long as it is a gluten free alternative, and there are a number of whole grains that will fit right into your diet, including rice. The best approach is to fill your home with gluten free foods first, and start cooking the things you love that revolve around them.

   Look online for gluten free recipes, and chat
with others in forums and chat rooms about what
they have learned along the way. In fact, once you
have adapted to the gluten free lifestyle, share
your ideas and solutions with others as well. It
certainly is not the easiest diet to conform to, so
any advice or suggestions are welcomed by all.

   Go to your local library and check out gluten
free cookbooks. When you get them home, scan the
recipes for foods you already have in the home, and
those you can add as a result of their suggestions.
Adapt the recipe as you see fit. If you do not like
tapioca, do not use it! Find another recipe that
does not contain it and move on. You do not have to
become a slave to the contents of recipes, you can
adapt them as you see fit as long as the foods you
are using are gluten free. As with any other diet,
cook what you like and you will be happy.

Eating out and on the go

   Eating outside of the home may seem tricky at
first, because you just do not know what to expect
from restaurants and their food preparation
efforts. Most restaurants willingly provide
vegetarian meals or even low fat alternatives, but
not everyone has caught on to the gluten free
approach to eating yet. The best course of action
in any restaurant is to make your server - and the
manager, if necessary - aware that you have a
gluten allergy. This will, hopefully, place the
kitchen on notice that when they are preparing your
food to use clean knives, cutting boards and pans
or skillets instead of a grill that may have
contained gluten-laced foods.

   Restaurants take food allergies very seriously,
whether you are at a large chain restaurant, or an
independently owned place. When you are looking for
gluten free foods on the menu, focus on vegetables

or lean meats. Make sure that whatever you order does not come with a "sauce" of any kind, and make it very clear to your server that your allergy will be affected as a result.

You do not have to be mean or forward with your requests, you must simply make the server aware that you absolutely cannot have your food contaminated by gluten products. In fact, ask for the manager and explain your condition to both of them at the same time – nicely. Afterwards, ask them for suggestions that may not be on the menu.

Often times there are vegetables or potatoes that are simply prepared plain, and sauces or toppings are added later. The staff can help you make wise choices, so trust them to lead you in the right direction. Also, look for things you know you can eat. If there is a steak sandwich on the menu ask for it without the bread. Avoid pastas, of course, and fried foods while scanning the menu for anything that works with your diet. Salad is a great alternative to guessing, so look for a green selection that fits - no dressing.

Choosing where to eat

You cannot always be in control of where you are going to eat, especially if you are enjoying a business lunch with colleagues or clients. However, if you know you are going to your best friend's favorite pizza place to celebrate their birthday in a couple of days, call ahead. Explain that you will be in soon, and that you would like to research their gluten free alternatives.

At times, the call ahead approach works brilliantly because you are not stunning the kitchen with your request when they are slammed with customers. The busier a place is, the more likely your requests are going to fall on deaf ears. However, if they know you are coming, they have time to prepare something on your behalf.

The truth is, you will be surprised by the number of restaurants that are catering to gluten free eaters these days, and are publishing their gluten free menus online.

The website, Gluten Free by Urban Tastebuds lists 75 (yes, the link says 68...but they have added to the list!) gluten free restaurant menus: http://www.glutenfreeguidehq.com/68-essential-gluten-free-restaurant-menus-you-need-to-know/

The list contains menus from fast food chains like Wendy's, McDonald's, Arby's and Chick-fil-a and chain restaurants like Applebee's, Hooters and Uno's Pizza (yes, pizza!). There are Italian and Mexican restaurants, seafood and steakhouses, as well as traditional options like burgers and chicken establishments. Check out the list, and work your outings around it if possible.

If you are going to a restaurant that is not on the list, call ahead and ask if they have a gluten free menu, or if they can prepare something for you. Be sincere, and kind, and ask to see the menu ahead of time so you can plan what you are going to eat on your own before you get there.

Do not be afraid to speak up about your gluten free preference. This is important, and can be completely accommodated without issue, as long as you ask!

Traveling

Traveling in a gluten free world means be careful about the things you eat. Much like the list above can help you find perfectly safe foods at home, you can also use it while you are traveling. In fact, research the restaurants in the area you are traveling to specifically for their gluten free offerings. You will be surprised by some of the awesome outlets that specialize in whole, organic, gluten free foods.

When you are on the go, whether you are flying, driving or taking the train, pack your own snacks so you can ensure there is always something safe to eat that is easily accessible. Packing nuts, an apple or banana will not only save you money, but it will provide you with a gluten free snack until you reach your destination.

Conclusion

Going gluten free means more than giving up bread. It means transforming your lifestyle to eat healthier, while keeping your digestive tract in check. If you legitimately have a gluten allergy or are even sensitive to its inclusion in foods, it is incredibly important that you abide by a complete gluten free diet to avoid damaging your body. This means never saying, "Oh, it will be fine to eat a sandwich" or "pasta, just this one time cannot hurt" because it can, and it will. Do not compromise your health simply to make your server's life easier.

Look for gluten free foods no matter where you are, and ensure that the label promises that is the case. Restaurants are more accommodating than ever to gluten free eating these days, and may even tout it on their menus, so look for those options where they are available. If they are not clear, ask your server or the manager. You certainly are not the first one who has requested a gluten free meal, and they will be glad to help you stay safe while dining with them.

Keep in mind that the world has changed, and that social media and restaurant review sites are very important to the livelihoods of restaurants and their staff. This is understood, so you should NEVER threaten a server or proprietor with a bad review. They already know that if they cannot accommodate your gluten free request, you are going to make it known to the world – which is why more and more establishments are following suit. It is not necessarily blackmail, but more of a good way to do business.

Devote your time and energy to becoming gluten free, as it takes dedication and commitment, especially if you are simply doing it for health reasons, and not because you have an allergy or reaction to eating foods that contain gluten. Research foods, recipes and healthier eating habits that will help you become gluten free as if it were second nature. Think about all of the good you are putting into your body, and stick to it. You really do not need pizza to live, and if so, the gluten free alternative is going to be tastier than you ever imagined!

Going gluten free is about finding out what is important to you, French fries and French dressing, or baked potatoes and balsamic vinegar? You will be amazed at how much better you feel, and how awakened your system will become when you stop eating gluten. Enjoy the healthier you, and help others in your home make better choices about what they eat as well. You are all going to want to see each other grow older, and going gluten free is a great way to maintain a steady, healthy diet while still enjoying the world around you.

Did you like this book?

I hope you learned a few things that will help you in your goals of either losing weight or just to eat healthier from my book.

I would really appreciate it if you would return to the Kindle store and leave a review and rating for this book, because Kindle rankings are driven by readers and customers like you.

I do hope you enjoyed this book and I would love to hear what you thought of it. You can leave your comments here:
http://www.amazon.com/dp/B00E66OLHW

Or you can simply go to Amazon.com and search for "**Start Living Gluten Free: A Beginners Guide to a Gluten Free Diet**", and this book's page will come up.

You May also be interested in other books I have done

The In's and Out's of Coconut Oil: A Beginners Guide

Modern Paleo Book 1: A Beginners Guide to the Paleo Diet

Modern Paleo Book 2: An Athletic Approach To The Paleo Diet

Book Bundles:

In's and Out's of Coconut Oil and Modern Paleo Beginner's Guide Book Bundle

Modern Paleo Book Bundle

The In's and Out's of Coconut Oil, Modern Paleo The Beginner's Guide and Athletic Approach Book Bundle

Thank you so much for purchasing my book.

Simone Donovan
http://simonedonovan.com/

www.ingramcontent.com/pod-product-compliance
Lightning Source LLC
Chambersburg PA
CBHW070823290526
45795CB00002B/824